Melba K. Haggins

Living in Our New Normal

Navigating from the shock of a diagnosis back to LIVING

Forward by Joseph C. Witherspoon, RRT

Copyright Page

Living In Our New Normal © Copyright *2021 Melba K Haggins*
All rights reserved. No part of this publication may be reproduced, distributed, or transmitted in any form or by any means, including photocopying, recording, or other electronic or mechanical methods, without the prior written permission of the publisher, except in the case of brief quotations embodied in critical reviews and specific other noncommercial uses permitted by copyright law.

Although the author and publisher have made every effort to ensure the information in this book was correct at press time, the author and publisher do not assume and hereby disclaim any liability to any party for any loss, damage, or disruption caused by errors or omissions, whether such errors or omissions result from negligence, accident, or any other cause. Adherence to all applicable laws and regulations, including international, federal, state, and local governing professional licensing, business practices, advertising, and all other aspects of doing business in the US, Canada, or any other jurisdiction, is the sole responsibility of the reader and consumer.

Neither the author nor the publisher assumes any responsibility or liability whatsoever on behalf of the consumer or reader of this material. Any perceived slight of any individual or organization is purely unintentional. **Physician names have been changed for privacy.**

The resources in this book are provided for informational purposes only and should not be used to replace the specialized training and professional judgment of a health care or mental health care professional. Neither the author nor the publisher can be held responsible for using the information provided within this book. Please always consult a trained professional before making any decision regarding the treatment of yourself or others.

For more information, email **info.melbashareshope@gmail.com**

Writing & Publishing Coaches: Cedric D. Nesbitt & Sinyon Shuntay

Editor: Venita D. Anderson

Cover Design: www.warriordesign.net

Library of Congress Control Number: 2021907757

ISBN: 978-1-7366488-0-3

10 9 8 7 6 5 4 3 2 1

Table of Contents

Dedication	i
Acknowledgments	ii
Foreword	iv
Preface	vi
Chapter 1 The Beginning of Different	1
Chapter 2 The Journey Begins	7
Chapter 3 A New World	14
Chapter 4 Training Days: Becoming a Caregiver	21
Chapter 5 Choosing a Home Healthcare Agency	27
Chapter 6 Coming Home!	31
Chapter 7 Welcoming Nurses into Your Home	41
Chapter 8 Navigating school – 504/Individual Education (IEP) Plans	48
Chapter 9 LIVE In Your New Normal	54
Develop Your Plan	64
References	69
About the Author	72

Dedication

I dedicate this book to God, my husband, Franklin, and children, Walter and Lydia. I am grateful to be living this life with you. This is not just my story; it is our story! I thank you for the gift of time, prayers, and grace to finish this God-given assignment. Walter, don't forget, you're an unstoppable warrior, and Lydia, you are beautiful sunshine. Franklin, you're the one. I love you all forever.

Acknowledgments

I first thank God for trusting Franklin and me to be Walter and Lydia's parents. Thank you for enabling us daily to LIVE our New Normal.

I thank God for my parents, Dorris & Milliard Freeman. Your memories are always with me and help me to stand.

I thank God for my mother-in-love, Frances 'Big Mama' Handberry, who loved us dearly. Our memories of you will never be forgotten.

I thank God for our natural and extended families. I thank God for each of you. Because of your love, support, and prayers, we have stood and still stand. Thank you for letting us just be. Mavis, my sister, and BFF thank you for everything. My bonus sons, daughter-in-love, and grandsons, I love you all dearly.

I want to thank every doctor and healthcare professional who has been a part of our healing journey.

A big THANK YOU to Walter's godparents, Willie & Ron Curry, who have stood by our sides through it all

Thank you to Lydia's godparents, Brian, Sr. & Janine Peacher, who stood with us and helped Walter have many playdates.

I thank our beloved Ms. Willie 'Ms.B.' Beard, who was a friend, another mom, and grandma to us. You helped to make Bloomington home for me. Your memory will forever be an imprint on my heart.

Thank you to my Pastors, Bishop Larry and Desetra Taylor, and my church family, Center For Hope International Ministries, who prayed for us, encouraged and supported us on this journey.

A special thanks to Char-Michelle McDowell for her encouragement during this book project. God did it!

Thank you, Mrs. Venita' Ms. V.' Anderson, for editing the book. Girl, you rock!

Thank you to my book writing tribe! You made the ride so much easier! Hats off to my coaches, Sinyon Shuntay and Cedric D. Nesbitt!

Thank you to my 100% Changed Leadership Edition Sisters for your prayers and encouragement!

If you said a prayer, sent a good thought or did a good deed, donated a gift card, money, or a meal, or shared an encouraging word during our journey, THANK YOU.

All GLORY to God for trusting me with this assignment and enabling me to complete it!

Foreword

"Your child needs a tracheostomy." These words, I wish no parent would ever hear. As a Respiratory Therapist with forty-plus years of experience with the last twelve years as Respiratory Coordinator of a pediatric tracheostomy and home ventilation program in a large Midwest children's hospital, I hear these words spoken all too often.

I first met Melba Haggins and her family during a routine visit to our clinic about a year after Walter's tracheostomy. From that time until his trach tube was permanently removed seven years later, I would see Walter and his family at least twice a year for check-ups.

I observed Walter as he grew into his teen years and was impressed by two of his qualities - the nearly normal teenage lifestyle he maintained and his extreme politeness. Walter hung out with friends, showed interest in playing sports and musical instruments. He did not let his tracheostomy hold him back. When he came in for check-ups, every question was answered with a "yes sir" or "no sir." This response was quite unusual for a teenager, especially these days. Both qualities I accredit to his parents, Melba and Franklin. They learned how to successfully incorporate his tracheostomy needs into a new normal lifestyle while maintaining the ability to be positive role models. This life experience uniquely qualifies Melba to provide the helpful information contained in this book.

I see the purpose of ***Living in Our New Normal*** as twofold. It will serve as a resource to other families with trach-dependent children by giving them hints to help their children live a high-quality life. Secondly, medical professionals and educators will use this book as a tool to help prepare families for daily life with a tracheostomy.

Joseph C. Witherspoon, RRT
Pediatric Pulmonology/Home Ventilation Program
Children's Hospital of Illinois
Peoria, IL

Preface

I've heard others talk about events in their lives that seem to take their breath away and totally sideswipe them. Well, my family had our first experience in 2007 when our lives were changed forever. My husband, Franklin, and I were working parents with two young children, Walter, six, and Lydia, eight months. On November 27, 2007, Walter had to have an emergency tracheotomy to help him breathe.

Our 'trach' journey began on that day. It radically changed our everyday life. We suddenly went from having, what we thought, was a healthy son, to one who had a life-threatening medical condition. We now had two children dependent on us in nearly *EVERY* way. There were medical terms, equipment, conditions, hospital stays, nurses, doctors, and nursing agencies. In addition to being parents, we were to become trained trach caregivers, advocates, employers, and social workers. All of this was in addition to the jobs we both held outside of the home. There was no guidebook, no Facebook group, nor support group to help us adjust or take in all of what this meant for our daily lives.

I hope this book will encourage families who have been blessed to love and care for a child with a critical medical condition. I will share a little of our journey, and at the end of the chapters, I will provide a few tips to help you on your journey. You will also have note pages at the end of the book to jot down information helpful for you. Please jot down questions, names, or ideas along the way. I want you to be able to determine how you will *live in your new normal.*

I hope sharing *Living In our New Normal*, will convince you that you are not alone, and will be a helpful resource for your family. May God bless you and your family as you 'LIVE in Your New Normal.'

Sincerely,

Melba K. Haggins

Chapter 1

The Beginning of Different

It was close to midnight on October 31, 2007, and there it was again — that croupy cough I had become accustomed to hearing. It seemed to occur more frequently after Walter started preschool. I had made a mental note to make him an appointment with the doctor the following morning. We heard this sound so many times; we knew exactly what it was. He was first diagnosed with croup around ten months old. We started albuterol nebulizer treatments at that time because the doctor thought he might be a borderline asthmatic. Walter was born eight weeks premature, and the doctor thought maybe this affected his lung development. Walter was now in first grade, full of energy, and taller than most of his classmates. I heard the coughing again. While I sat finishing my work on the computer, I made another mental note to call the doctor the next morning.

I heard it again; this time, something was different. I rushed to Walter's room as he was still coughing. He was awake and said, "Mom, I don't feel too good,"... and suddenly, with one gag, emptied all his stomach contents onto his sheets. My mother's intuition was kicking in hard and saying this was not normal. I proceeded to get him, and his bed cleaned up and told him we were going to the emergency room. I rushed to get everything ready, called my husband, who worked the graveyard shift at our local hospital, to meet us. I carefully bundled up our sleeping baby girl and headed to the hospital's emergency room. Franklin met us at the emergency room and took Walter inside. I drove around the corner to Mom Willie's house, who was both grandma and babysitter, to drop Lydia off to continue her night's sleep. Afterwards, I immediately returned to join Walter and Franklin.

They kept Walter in the emergency room overnight, treating him with an albuterol nebulizer and steroid treatments at regular intervals, but he didn't improve. This resulted in him being hospitalized before breakfast that morning. Walter was stable, but still not much improvement. I left the hospital late afternoon to pick our baby daughter up from daycare and bring her by the hospital for a quick visit. After visiting, we went home, and my husband stayed with Walter at the hospital.

After feeding Lydia and putting her down for the evening, I received a call. It was the hospital. A woman's voice on the phone asked for me and asked me if someone could bring me to the hospital.

I stiffened. "WAIT a minute, I need you to tell me what's going on!"

She said, "Walter is in respiratory failure. He stopped breathing."

"I will be there. I will drive myself."

I steadied myself and hung up. "Stay calm."

I just knew I had to remain calm to get everything done. I started praying. I called Mom Willie to let her know and to see if she could keep Lydia. She would meet me at the hospital. After getting Lydia's things together, we were off.

I drove and prayed while the tears forced themselves down my face. Crying was the last thing I needed. I needed to focus. Focus on the God Promise over my son's life. I felt that promise was the only thing that could keep everything together. I had to hold onto it with everything I had to fight the wild panic that was threatening to overcome me. I called a friend from church to let her know what was happening and to pray. I continued to busy myself praying and reminding God of His promises as I drove. I declared Walter would live and not die. We made it to the hospital, and Mom Willie arrived at the same time. I handed Lydia over to her and zoomed upstairs to Walter's hospital room.

He was lying flat as a board on the bed, not moving, not breathing. An army of doctors and nurses surrounded his bed.

My husband was in the far corner on the opposite side of the room. The Priest was at the door. Everybody was in panic mode, giving Walter all of their attention. I felt like I was caught in a horror movie happening before my eyes. They were working to save Walter and to get him back breathing. The Respiratory Tech was practically in tears.

I couldn't just stand there! Just as suddenly as I entered the room, I left the room, pushing past the Priest. I didn't want to see the Priest because no last rites were going to be read that night. He moved to ask me a question, and I held my hand up- no, not now.

I went to the lobby to breathe and pray. I called my brother, the Patriarch of our bunch, to tell him. Then the tears came freely without restraint, down my face. I got off the phone with him and went back to the room. A few minutes later, Walter had a shallow breath; they bagged him and began to prepare him for medical transport to the Children's Hospital of Illinois in Peoria, which was about 45 minutes from our home.

The doctor called my husband and me in for a consultation. Walter was transported on a Life Flight to the Children's Hospital of Illinois' Pediatric Intensive Care Unit (PICU). He told us to take our time, to get clothes, and everything else we needed because they would have to connect Walter in PICU before we could see him anyway. We rushed home, packed some clothes and extra things for the baby. We took Lydia to Mom Willie's and headed to Peoria.

Oh my God! There were so many tubes, cords, and machines on Walter, it was overwhelming. I thought, is he alive, or is the machine breathing for him? He was in an induced coma. The intubation tube they used in the prior hospital was too large and had scraped the inside of his esophagus. His esophagus was raw inside, and they had to suction the blood-tainted fluid from that injury as well. What caused all of this? Our journey had begun!

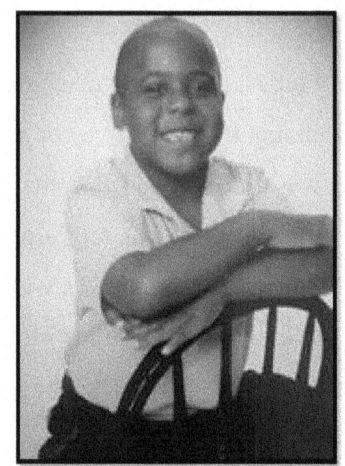
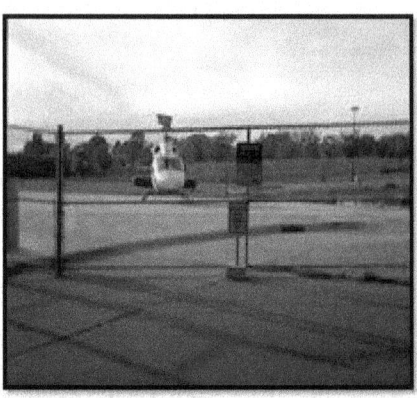

*The
Beginning of Different*

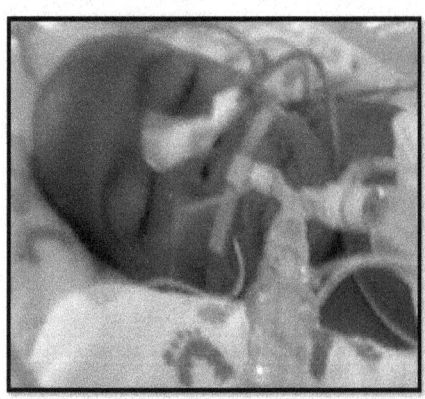

Chapter 2

The Journey Begins

As I stood there beside Walter's PICU bed looking at him lying there lifeless with all of the tubes and the machines connected, beeping and blinking colored lights, I wondered if my baby boy would actually make it. When I looked up, I noticed a Minister from our church had arrived and was standing in the doorway. She caught my eye and said to me,

"It is well. Look at me! It is well."

The words seemed to bring calm to my soul. It was the confirmation I needed to help me remain calm and continue to believe.

The questions came-when did it start? Does Walter have asthma? How long had he been on breathing treatments? Was he full-term or prematurely born? There were tests on top of tests. Initial tests showed he had an infection in his trachea, which I believed came from the life-saving techniques. The doctors began to treat Walter with antibiotics and continued to give him albuterol nebulizer treatments. Walter's breathing didn't improve much, but then they added steroid breathing treatments, which seemed to help. He was moved out of PICU to a step-down floor four days later after he had responded well to the steroid treatments. The doctors ordered a CT scan (3-D X-ray) to get a closer look at Walter's airway. They had to intubate him because he was nervous and afraid during the scan. After a couple of days of being on the regular floor, he was released from the hospital with prescriptions and instructions for a steady breathing treatment regimen and steroids. Walter was in the hospital a week which seemed long and short at the same time. It was too long to be afraid of losing my son, yet short in the sense that everything seemed to have happened so fast. We were glad to be going home, but it still seemed like I was holding my breath because I knew they didn't have the root cause.

A few days later, the Saturday after his release, I heard Walter again. His breathing was very loud and labored. I could hear every inhaled breath. We called the pediatrician, who asked us to bring him into the office. My husband took Walter to the doctor's office while I stayed home with Lydia. Soon after, my husband called to let me know Walter was going back to the Children's Hospital of Illinois in Peoria. This time, he was sent by ambulance. My husband rode along with Walter. I packed some clothes for them and headed over.

Here we go again, more tests and treatments, but no real answers. The doctor told us a child with a normal airway shouldn't have croup after four years old, and it should manifest more like hoarseness or laryngitis as a child gets older. That had not been the case for Walter. We knew something was not right. Walter was released after about five days just before Thanksgiving with a follow-up appointment for a CT scan. The doctors wanted to get a better look at Walter's airway in its natural state and asked us to help him be relaxed for the CT scan.

On Thursday, November 29, 2007, we drove to Peoria for the 10 am CT scan. We continued to encourage Walter not to be afraid of the CT scan and help the doctor get a good picture. We told him it was like a big camera, and we needed him to lay quietly for the scan. He did wonderfully! We ate lunch and waited for our 1 pm follow-up with the doctor for the results.

We met Dr. Vagu in his office. He asked were we able to get the CT scan completed okay. We assured him we did, and he left the room to check the results. After only a few minutes, he rushed back into the room and asked us to follow him to see the results. I was a bit alarmed inside as I sensed an element of urgency in his voice. We hurried and gathered our belongings, but he said we could leave our coats in the office. We rushed out and followed him. We entered another room where there was a computer monitor with Walter's CT scan results. We saw the results in a 3-D fashion. He showed us the pathway from Walter's mouth down through his airway. **Walter's airway was blocked in the larynx area!** There was only a tiny opening, about the size of the tip of a writing pen.

I gasped. **OH MY GOD**, what was blocking my son's airway?!

Dr. Vagu said he couldn't tell what it was. He would need to take Walter to surgery.

He led us back to his office. That walk back was like an out-of-body experience....in shock, fear, trying to stay calm, and praying all the way there. A portion of scripture came to my mind, *speak to the mountain,* as I made it back to the office door. Dr. Vagu explained that he couldn't let us take Walter home. Walter was in trouble because the small airway he had could close at any moment. **WALTER NEEDED AN EMERGENCY TRACHEOTOMY to help him breathe.** He instructed us to immediately admit Walter to PICU to get him ready for surgery as soon as possible.

My brain was overwhelmed at the thought Walter could have died in his sleep or even on the car ride to the hospital. I was grateful to God for His protection. Walter had slept with me the previous night, and I was up nearly all night listening to and for his breathing. I heard the loud, labored breathing as he slept. Was this happening? What was blocking his airway? Many thoughts and emotions were running through my head and body, too much to make sense of it all. The main thing was to be strong and help Walter navigate what was happening. Walter was all that mattered now.

Walter was admitted to PICU, and we waited in the room with him. All Walter wanted was the Nintendo machine so he could play games. They brought it, and that kept him occupied while we waited for surgery. Walter went to surgery around 7 pm, and we waited some more.

Dr. Vagu came out to speak with us after Walter's surgery was completed. He explained the surgery went well, and Walter's vocal cords were actually blocking his airway and not moving to allow him to breathe as needed. Also, Dr. Vagu shared there was some type of crystallization on Walter's vocal cords, and they didn't know what it was. They were running additional tests to determine what it may be. My mind started to race. *Did my baby have cancer or something else awful? What were we to expect? A trach and cancer, Lord?!*

I said to myself, "Melba, snap out of it and believe all will be well." It was so much, and it was happening so fast. It was as if I was on autopilot.

They brought Walter back to the room, and he was still asleep. I briefly flashbacked to the prior two weeks as I looked at the tubes and machines connected to Walter. I felt a lump in my throat for a few minutes and that feeling like I was holding my breath as I stood by his bed. There were those plugs, cords, tubes, and machines. Now this trach tube was in his neck. *Would my baby be able to talk? Would he need some device to be able to speak? What does this mean? Would he be able to eat by mouth? How do we take care of him? How long will he need this trach thing? And what's on his vocal cords?* So many questions in my mind, and I didn't have the answers. In my mind, I remembered this man I'd seen, when I was little, in the grocery store who'd put this thing up to his neck so he could talk to the clerk. Would my son be like that; robot-like talking while holding this device to his neck?

At last, Walter woke up; and again, all he wanted was the Nintendo remote control. That was his pacifier, and he played until he drifted back to sleep. Nursing was around the clock, and so were we. The nurses were regularly suctioning secretions from Walter's trach tube. With the trach, his ability to cough up mucus was reduced because of the airway's opening. I was relieved Walter seemed to be relaxed. However, my mind was wondering what was next?

What is a Tracheostomy?

A tracheotomy is an opening surgically created through the neck into the trachea (windpipe) to allow direct access to the lungs. A tracheostomy tube, commonly called a trach tube, is usually placed through this opening to provide an airway and to suction secretions from the lungs. The opening is called a stoma. With a tracheostomy, breathing is done through the trach tube rather than through the nose and mouth.

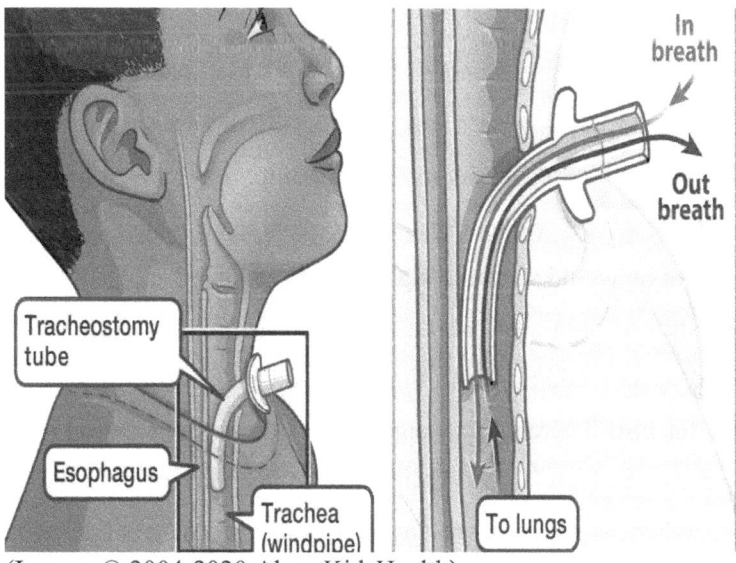
(Image: © 2004-2020 AboutKidsHealth)

Chapter 3

A New World

The answers began to come. Walter should be able to talk. His body would have to get accustomed to the different paths of his airflow. But Walter wasn't saying anything, only moved his lips, mouthed words, and pointed. We encouraged Walter to try to talk, but he would start to cough every time he did. The coughing made him afraid to try. Walter needed to stay in the hospital for a while so he could adjust to the trach and for us to learn how to care for him. There was no answer for how long he would need the trach. As far as the crystallization on his vocal cords, some of the preliminary tests were negative and more tests were being done. In the meantime, the PICU Lead doctor, Dr. Terry worked to get us an appointment with one of the top otolaryngologist doctors in the U.S. either in Chicago or Cincinnati, to do further testing and consultation on Walter's airway. We prayed for Chicago as Cincinnati would be more than a notion for travel.

Walter moved from PICU to the ward, which was like the next level of care down from PICU. He still had nursing around the clock. My husband and I decided to be around the clock too. Franklin took a Family Medical Leave of Absence (FMLA) from work and stayed with Walter at the hospital. I stayed home to keep the baby on a regular schedule and to work as much as possible. I traveled back and forth to the hospital, which was forty-five minutes from our home.

I stayed the first Friday night after Walter was moved to the new ward to give my husband a break and allow him to get everything ready for the extended stay. I talked to Walter about trying to speak with the trach and encouraged him to keep trying. I assured him the coughs would stop as his body got used to breathing differently. **And then it happened! He tried to speak again! He spoke his first words with the trach! His first Breakthrough! He kept talking!!**

The only thing now was that I couldn't hear my baby laugh or cry. The tracheostomy did not allow enough air to flow over the vocal cords to make a strong sound. You never know how much those sounds mean to you. Would I ever hear his chuckling jolly laugh again? His whole face lit up when he laughed. I smiled, just thinking about his jolly laugh.

Next, Walter was moved to the tracheostomy ward, room G214. We were becoming very familiar with The Children's Hospital of Illinois. He shared G214 with four other children, three of whom were trach-dependent, and one recently had his trach removed. These were children of all ages – infants through teens. A whole new world! G214 would now be a home away from home.

Then, Dr. Terry informed us it was time for another temporary move. He had gotten Walter an appointment with Dr. Hollins in Chicago on December 10, 2007, for further consultation and diagnosis. Thankfully, all testing of the crystallization on his vocal cords was negative – but still a mystery. Walter would be transported by ambulance to Lurie Children's Hospital in Chicago. Franklin would ride in the ambulance with Walter. I made it over to Peoria that morning and saw Walter and Franklin off as they prepared for the ambulance ride to Chicago. It kind of stung because I really wanted to go be there with them.

I informed our Pastors, Bishop Larry and Elder Desetra Taylor, they were in Chicago, and the doctor had planned to take Walter to surgery the next day to take a look.

Bishop asked, "You want to be there, don't you?"

"Yes," I confessed.

He had his assistant purchase a train ticket for me. I looked on Lurie Children's website and noticed the hospital had a shuttle bus to the train station. I was relieved and excited because I wouldn't have to worry about navigating from the Chicago train station. This was my first train ride to Chicago, and I was elated to be with my son for his surgery. I left the baby with her grandma for the overnight stay. I was so happy; God had answered the desires of my heart!

Franklin didn't tell Walter I was coming. When I stepped into the hospital room, Walter was extremely excited.

"Mom," he yelled as much as he could. "I didn't know you were coming!"

We hugged like we hadn't seen each other in months.

We met Dr. Hollins, a tall, slim, older gentleman. He was very professional, personable, and a sincere doctor. He did a couple of magic tricks with Walter to break the ice. Dr. Hollins would take him to surgery for a bronchoscopy to look at his airway and possibly remove some tissue for further testing. He was a top-notch doctor in his field; after all, his father invented a trach tube. We felt God had aligned our steps, and we were where we needed to be.

We also met the doctor's nurse, who was a real hoot. She had us complete the necessary paperwork for Walter and gave us some good advice too. She worked with multiple trach children and their families, so she had the inside scoop. We were like two sponges, soaking it all up. Her talk seemed to relieve a burden and the fear of the unknown that I was seemingly bravely bearing. She encouraged us to continue to parent and not to be soft on Walter because of his trach. She told us how children sometimes would act to avoid discipline.

She said, "That trach won't come out!"

At this point, we just knew Walter couldn't breathe independently, he needed this trach tube, and we couldn't bring him home. We didn't know the root cause or how long it would be before he could come home. We didn't understand what we needed to do. The nurse's chat was just what we needed. It was like getting a fresh breath of air, awakened from a nightmare, back to reality, where we could hear and have hope there was life ahead.

Walter went to surgery, and we waited to find out what the diagnosis would be. After, Dr. Hollins said the surgery went well, and it seemed the crystallization on his vocal cords was caused by acid reflux. He suggested Dr. Terry perform further testing and put Walter on acid reflux medication immediately. It was good to have an answer for the crystallization on the vocal cords, and know it was not some other horrible disease attacking my son's body.

I took the hospital shuttle back to the Chicago train station to head back home after Walter's surgery and consultation with the doctors. Walter and Franklin were taken back to Peoria the following day by ambulance to continue their stay. Walter's attending physician, Dr. Terry, put Walter on a low dose of acid reflux medication but didn't do further testing. The saga continued in G214. We had entered a whole new world.

Tips: Preparing for a Dr. Visit or Consultation

When you're going to consult with a new doctor or follow up on results from testing or complicated medication situations, here are some tips to follow.

- Bring a notepad/pen or electronic device to take notes and jot down questions. Also, bring questions you may already have.
- Take a list of your current prescription and over the counter medications and vitamins.
- If you can, ask a family member or friend to accompany you so he or she can ask questions or remember items you may miss.
- Speak up if you don't understand. There are no dumb questions. This is not the time to be shy.
- Be an advocate! If the proposed treatment doesn't seem right, ask for alternatives.
- If treatment doesn't seem to be getting to the root issue, ask what else can be done to determine the cause and prevent a repeat.
- Always ask how and who you can follow up with for additional questions you may have later.
- Get the contact information for the doctors and any assistants who meet with you.
- Request that any necessary blood work/tests be ordered before your check-up appointments. This eliminates extra appointments and allows you the opportunity to review results during your upcoming visit.

Keep a calendar of prior/upcoming doctor appointments, surgeries, and procedures. The calendar will be a helpful record, so you don't have to remember everything on the spot. I wrote everything on the calendar; then, I have a history of each visit at the end of the year. Just know, after a while, you will sound like a broken record to yourself, repeating the same medical information over and over. I kept all pictures and documents of everything in a file. It was a good thing. After all, one of his doctors asked me if I had saved his prior surgery pictures because some had not been transferred after upgrading the hospital's computer system. I was able to fax her copies.

Chapter 4

Training Days: Becoming a Caregiver

We were now almost three weeks into this journey. Walter was still in the hospital, yet we hadn't learned how to take care of him. We would become more than parents; we would now need to be trained trach nurses. Our duties and responsibilities would be expanded. Would we be able to care for him? What would it mean for our home, life, and his school?

I had been traveling to the hospital nearly every day of the week. I regularly spent Sunday afternoons, Monday, Wednesday, and Friday evenings at the hospital, along with any other specific days I needed or wanted to be there. During the week, I would get Lydia and myself ready in the mornings. I'd then drop her off at her grandma and arrive at my office by 8 am. At work, I was leading and managing a team daily. I would leave work, pick up Lydia, and then head to the hospital. We usually made it to the hospital around 5:30 pm, stayed a couple of hours, and was back home by 9 pm. My sister jokingly said my van could probably automatically drive itself to Peoria because of our regular trips. It was a full schedule, but somehow, I don't remember feeling tired. This was what needed to be done at that time. God had given me the grace I needed for the situation.

We finally were told the training days were going to start. One step closer to home! The training days were Monday and Thursday evenings. I adjusted my regular hospital visiting schedule to go over for training days and Fridays. I would leave the baby with her grandma or her godmother on some training nights before heading to the hospital for class. The training class was Walter's hospital room. Walter's godmother rode with me on most training nights to learn how to care for Walter right along with us. After training started, I decided to stay home on the weekends. This allowed time for others to visit and for me to get some downtime. I spent time with our growing baby girl, and of course, getting the regular household stuff done – washing, cleaning, paying bills, and all the things that never stop. It also gave me a chance to connect with my church's women's group and fellowship.

We had Nurse Colleen, the respiratory nurse from the Vent clinic, training us to care for Walter. We were to learn what a tracheostomy was, how to recognize respiratory distress, how to change Walter's trach, and do daily cleaning and care. We had to learn about the equipment and how to operate and maintain it. We had to learn proper suctioning techniques, both sterile and non-sterile. We even had to learn how to do CPR for a tracheostomy. Wow, this training was for life- the most critical class I'd ever taken. It was real and practical training with an actual patient, my firstborn son. He was probably just as nervous as we were but was a true champion. Walter would only allow his dad and me to touch his trach tube. He would not let anyone else change the trach tube, and that never changed. He held it in place when we did the cleaning and changed the trach ties. Walter was his own trach police.

At this point, we were willing to do just about anything to get Walter back home. I felt if we could get home, it would be better. It was day to day and week to week learning and becoming proficient in the various trach care procedures and equipment. I think we could have earned college credits for this training.

Tips: Recognizing Respiratory Distress

The first thing we learned was how to recognize respiratory distress, as this could be a sign to us that Walter needed suctioning or that something was blocking his trach tube. We also learned how to perform CPR (Cardiopulmonary resuscitation) for a child with a tracheostomy.

People with trouble breathing often show signs that they have to work harder to breathe or are not getting enough oxygen, indicating respiratory distress. Below is a list of some of the signs that may indicate a person is working harder to breathe and may not be getting enough oxygen. It is essential to learn the signs of respiratory distress to know when your child may need immediate care.

- **Breathing rate.** An increase in the number of breaths taken per minute may mean a person is having trouble breathing or not getting enough oxygen.
- **Color changes.** A bluish color around the mouth, inside the lips, or fingernails may happen when a person is not getting the needed oxygen. The color of the skin may also appear pale or gray.
- **Grunting.** If a grunting sound can be heard each time the person exhales, that's the body's way of trying to keep the air in the lungs so they will stay open.

- **Nose flaring.** The nostrils of the nose spreading open while breathing may mean a person has to work harder to breathe.
- **Retractions.** The chest appears to sink in just below the neck or under the breastbone with each breath or both. This is one way of bringing more air into the lungs and can also be seen under the rib cage or even in the ribs' muscles.
- **Sweating.** There may be increased sweat on the head, but the skin does not feel warm to the touch. More often, the skin may feel cool or clammy. This may happen when the breathing rate is very fast.
- **Wheezing.** A tight, whistling, or musical sound heard with each breath can mean that the air passages may be smaller (tighter), making it harder to breathe.
- **Body position.** A person may spontaneously lean forward while sitting to help take deeper breaths. This is a warning sign that he or she is about to collapse.

Your doctor or hospital most likely will provide you information on how to do daily trach care and maintenance. Please refer to any specific information for your child's particular needs. There are also several resources on the internet that will detail how to do the daily care of the trach and stoma area and how to change the trach tube.

Just remember, cleanliness is imperative to your child's health. Make sure your hands and all caregiver's hands are washed thoroughly before doing any trach care or suctioning. Keep the trach supplies in a location where they can stay dry and clean. Equipment and supplies should be kept clean to keep germs, dust, and dirt away. Follow all necessary safety protocols and don't cut corners.

Chapter 5

Choosing a Home Healthcare Agency

It was now time to choose a nursing agency to care for Walter. We were getting closer as we checked things off the list for going home. ***Walter was considered a medically fragile child because the only thing standing between life and death for him was the trach tube. He would need to be with a trained caregiver at all times.*** My husband and I worked outside of the home. We needed nursing care for him during those times. I worked days, and Franklin worked the night shift.

Choosing a home healthcare agency was probably one of the scariest things on the list because I had to accept the reality that our lives were changing for real. I wondered how in the world we would pay for this stuff in the back of my mind. We already had two mortgages as we closed on a new home to make room for the baby before selling our old house, and we didn't have any buyer prospects for our old home. We had health insurance, but how much would that cover? My thoughts would swing from contemplating the cost to wondering how it would work to have nurses in our home every day. Wow, this was more than a notion. It was a different world.

I remember going through the telephone book and looking for home health agencies. I had no idea about any of them and hadn't heard of most. I may have seen commercials about a couple of them, but they were focused on senior citizens. I asked other parents about the nursing agencies they were using and got some clues. I was able to get about three names, and that's where I started my search. I called each agency and began to ask the questions I wanted and needed to know. I got through most of my questions with a couple of the agencies, but for the most part, I would sense after the first few questions whether to pursue. Some of the questions I asked were:

- Are you currently serving any trach-dependent children?
- Are your nurses trained on tracheostomy care? How do they receive training? Is there ongoing training?
- How much experience do you have working with children?
- What areas/cities do you serve? How far do your nurses travel?
- What happens if there is no nurse availability? What do you do to get coverage?
- Do you currently or have you served Black/African American families/children? (This was new to me, and Walter was the only Black child in the room. I wanted to know my family wasn't the only family.)

I was very direct and honest with my questions because my child's life depended on proper care. I could not afford to get it wrong right out of the gate.

After a few days, I had finally narrowed it down to two nursing agencies. They both were serving trach-dependent children and had nurses working in our area at that time. What made the difference was the sense of peace I had with the nursing agency we chose. The owner had told me about the company's history and their passion for the service they provided. She talked about how she considered the children and families as part of their extended family. They even held specific events to provide opportunities to gather with all the families to celebrate. The owner took her time and was patient while I went down my list of questions. I felt they would be more responsive to our needs. Also, they had served African American children, which was a big plus in my book.

This was another check on our prerequisite checklist for leaving the hospital. We had now chosen a nursing agency.

Tips: Choosing a Home Healthcare Agency

The main things I wanted from a home healthcare agency were professionalism, trach experience, and sufficient staff to cover our needed hours. I wanted an agency that was personable and where it didn't seem like we were just another case, but a family. I chose our healthcare agency because of those reasons and because they had experienced staff available to care for Walter as needed. Here are some tips for you as you search for a home healthcare agency.

- Look up the agency on the BBB (Better Business Bureau) site and google the name to see if there are negative complaints. If so, are they consistently around some of the same services?
- Do they have trained staff? How are they trained? Are there continuing education opportunities for nurses on tracheostomy care?
- Will they be able to cover your hours/needs? Or will you need to hire additional help?
- If a nurse isn't a good fit, what do you need to do to get a replacement?
- If your regular nurse is ill or unavailable, do they provide coverage/substitute?
- What care should you expect the nurses to provide for your child?
- If there are scheduling changes, how are those communicated?
- What do you need to provide in your home to accommodate the nurse?

Chapter 6

Coming Home!

We were putting the pieces together, learning to care for Walter, operating the medical equipment, and decoding the medical terminology. We knew how to recognize respiratory distress, do daily trach cleaning, safely suction, change the tracheostomy tube, and work the equipment- the essential requirements to keep Walter safe. We had even chosen a home healthcare agency. We were getting closer to home.

We celebrated Christmas and New Year's in the hospital. I bought a little tabletop Christmas tree for Christmas and decorated it for Walter's hospital room area. Walter was ecstatic about Christmas! Many kind and thoughtful people donated gifts and toys to encourage the children in the hospital, and Walter loved every minute of it! It was a blessing to experience the love and concern from others. The Child Life Specialist asked Walter what he wanted for Christmas. That year he asked for a Transformer and an Electronic Hyper Slide. Well, Santa searched all over for the Hyper Slide and finally located one. Walter got his wish! The memory of that day was captured forever in my heart and the local newspaper.

We finally got a target date for home, January 18, 2008. That was like music in our ears. After all, Walter had been hospitalized since November 29, 2007. Franklin had been with him daily, and I'd been traveling back and forth, working, and caring for Lydia. It would be good for everybody to be home.

I had to get Walter's room ready at home for the additional equipment that would become a staple in his room and make room for the nurse to be there. Wow, this would mean no more of Walter sneaking into our bedroom at night. The nurse's home base would mainly be in his room. I hoped we would like the nurse, and the nurse would like us too. But those worries faded away at the thought and pleasure of having Walter back home in his own bed. We would do what was necessary to keep him safe, and that's what mattered.

A girlfriend from church came over and helped me get everything rearranged in Walter's room. We moved a desk and desk chair from the basement to Walter's room to have a place for the nurse to use while in his room. We made space on each side of his bed for equipment. I bought portable storage bin carts to store his trach supplies to keep them organized and clean. It was like getting ready to bring a new baby home for the first time. I felt the same anticipation as I did when I brought the 11-

day old, 4lb 3oz preemie home for the first time. We were making room.

Then we hit a snag....coming home could be delayed. I had asked our pediatrician about having our daughter tested to see if she had any issues. He had previously expressed some concern about her breathing after hearing her sleeping when we came in for one of her appointments. He listened to a slight rattling sound coming from her and asked, did she always sound like that when she slept? He checked her, and the sound was located in her throat area. I remembered that. We had already experienced the whirlwind with Walter, so I wanted a closer look at Lydia and a check for any acid reflux issues. Her pediatrician ordered a bronchoscopy with a gastric reflux test. It was set for January 7, 2008, 11 days from Walter's scheduled release date. She would have to stay overnight in the hospital for the gastric reflux test to be monitored. Our whole family was in the same hospital due to Lydia's test. I stayed with Lydia overnight, and Franklin was in his regular place with Walter. Lydia's room was up the hall on the opposite side of the floor from Walter's room.

The results came in the following day. Lydia had a slight abnormality in her airway, nothing to be concerned about right then but to watch. She also had some acid reflux. Because her test was positive for acid reflux, I asked Dr. Terry to have Walter tested for acid reflux. He did.

Oh boy, Walter's acid reflux was at the top of the charts. His acid reflux came all the way up to his throat. **Finally, we'd found the culprit! Acid Reflux really was the nemesis!** Now we fully understood why the crystallization was on his vocal cords. We had the test results to show it. Acid reflux had scarred his larynx area and caused his vocal cords to be fixed in place, blocking his airway. Now what?

Dr. Terry was amazed at Walter's test results. The diagnosis we received from Chicago was on point. Dr. Terry now wanted to keep Walter in the hospital a little longer to perform a procedure that would reduce the acid escaping from his stomach. We were disappointed as this would lengthen Walter's hospital stay for at least three more weeks. Fortunately, Nurse Colleen convinced the doctor to allow him to come home as planned and schedule Walter's stomach procedure out 3-4 weeks later. **We were back on schedule**! I was relieved to know we would all be under one roof again soon. This schedule allowed enough time to learn about and plan the upcoming procedure.

Coming Home Day had arrived! Walter would be transported home in an ambulance with our training nurse accompanying him. Franklin would follow behind in his truck. I was home on pins and needles, waiting for Franklin's call to let me know they were on their way. I took the day off work, and I was just home nesting like a mother-to-be getting ready for her newborn baby. There were balloons on the mailbox. I had a big sign in the foyer welcoming Walter home! I had lunch cooked and ready. Walter's room was perfect for him and his new equipment. The house was clean and prepared for my babies– Walter and Franklin. I got the call! They were on their way…in 45 minutes, my Walter would be home!

The ambulance pulled up in the driveway, and I bum-rushed the door with cheerleader pom-poms in hand! Walter rushed out past the nurse as quickly as he could and nearly tackled me with the best hug ever! Tears of joy flowed down my face as I embraced him. I looked up, and the nurse was in tears too. We were all so happy and overjoyed Walter was finally home. The nurse checked out Walter's room, got him set-up, took his vitals, and left us to ourselves. We were all back under the same roof. Thank You, Lord!!

Tips: Preparing for your home life

Being ready for home-life requires preparation and organization. It will take longer to prepare for the day and bed, so having a regular schedule that everyone knows will help tremendously. We had standard awake times, baths, and bedtimes.

To leave home, we had to have a suction bag and an emergency bag with all of the necessary equipment to keep Walter safe in case of an emergency. In Walter's emergency bag, we carried the following:

- Ambu bag
- An extra sterile trach tube
- Sterile trach tube ½ size smaller
- Sterile catheters w/sterile gloves
- Powder-free gloves
- Scissors
- Suction tips
- Saline solution (pinkies)
- 6-inch swabs
- Split gauze pads
- Trach ties
- KY Gel
- Vaseline

Everywhere we went with Walter, we had the two bags. We also always kept another emergency bag packed in his room in case of emergency so that we always knew there was a bag ready if needed.

Medical Supply List: Trach/Medical supplies will need to be ordered each month. It will be a good idea to make a list or a copy of the required supplies list so that you can easily order what is needed each month and track your orders. Usually, Walter's day nurse would make the monthly order; however, we also had to make orders sometimes. It is easier to track when there is a standard list. I kept a list on my computer to print off and mark up each month. Always consult your doctor for your particular equipment needs.

Here's a sample of Walter's trach supply list.

	Trach Supply List		
	Month	Date Ordered	
Product Description	Manufacturer	Model #	Quantity
Suction Machine	Devilbiss		
Suction Machine	Devilbiss		
Air Compressor			
Pulse Oximeter			
O2 system			
The Vest			
Heater - wrap around			
Oxygen Bulb			
Suction canister	Benis	2130-8002CP	2
Suction filter	Devilbiss	17305D608	2
Suction elbow	Devilbiss	17305D023	2
Suction Tubing 6'	Cardinal	N56A	2
Sterile Suction Catheter 10 FR	Care Fusion	4865T	60
Oral Suction Catheter (pink top)	Kimberly-Clark	1222	4
Trach Tube Bivona 4.0	Bivona		1
Trach Tube Bivona 3.5	Bivona		
Trach Tube Ties	Dale 240	H8410**240**	30
Trach mask	Care Fusion	1225	1
Corrigated tubing (blue tube)		1680	1 box
Water Trap	Cardinal	001860	2
Large Volume Nebulizer	Hudson	1770	2
Valved Tee Adapter	Cardinal	2060	
Nebulizer Kit	Salter Labs	8900	1
Nebulizer mask	Cardinal	1263	1
Thermovent t's	Smiths Medical	570016	60
Pulse Oximeter Probes	Masimo SET	LNCS Neo-L	4
Q-Tips	Kendall	541400	2 boxes
Sorb-it Drain Sponges 4x4	Kendall	6242P	2 boxes
Sterile NaCl (pinkies)	AddiPak	200-39	2 boxes
Tape (Transpore)	3M		1 box
Oxygen Tubing 25'	B & F Medical	64232	
Oxygen Tubing 7'	Cardinal	1302	
Specimen Trap (40 ml)	Kendall	724500	

Special Numbers List: Keeping an updated list of important numbers in an easily accessible place will be very helpful. Your nurse or nursing agency may ask for it. In Walter's room, we had a list of important numbers and information posted above the desk near the telephone. We included our work and cell numbers, our emergency contacts' cell and home phones, and Walter's physicians' contact numbers. We listed every emergency number from 911 to the Insurance Company's number. At that time, we had to have a landline because of the 911 service. You will need to check with your area if that is necessary.

Special Services: Because your child will have special needs in case of an emergency, there are certain services you may qualify for and register to receive. Most will require you to complete specific paperwork about your child's medical needs. Because Walter had durable medical equipment critical to his health requiring electricity, our home was put on the durable equipment list with our electric company. This put our house on the top of the list in case of a power outage. The only alternative was to go to the hospital. Also, our county had special services for those with critical medical conditions to allow them to get to and receive necessary emergency care in hazardous weather. Our neighborhood street was always cleared of snow as a priority to make it easier for us in emergencies. Our nearest fire department was also notified about my son's medical condition and made aware of the oxygen tanks in our home in case of a fire emergency.

We also had to have an emergency plan posted in case of fire and a fire extinguisher and working fire and carbon monoxide alarms.

Chapter 7

Welcoming Nurses into Your Home

Having a nurse, really a stranger, in our home was a foreign concept for us to take in. On the one hand, I was glad to have support, but on the other hand, a stranger would be in my personal, private space. Growing up in my household, one of the things I heard was, *"What happens in the house, should stay in the house. Don't put your business out in the streets."*

I didn't want my family's business part of the daily news. These thoughts were rambling through my head, and I had to let them go.

Walter's first day nurse was perfect for getting us accustomed to our 'new normal'. She was experienced, helpful, and on top of that, Walter liked her, and we did too. We had full nursing coverage for school, 7 am - 4 pm M-F, to allow Walter to go to school safely while I worked, and Franklin slept. At night, we had coverage at 10 pm – 7 am to let me sleep while Franklin worked. This schedule also allowed us to have our family time daily from 4-10 pm during the week without a nurse. On the weekends, we only had night coverage. This schedule allowed the flexibility for us to have dinner together and time to bond as a family. We were still able to get Walter and Lydia ready for bed and do the everyday things. When the nurse came at night, Walter was generally in bed already or preparing for bed. The night nurse's main job was to monitor him through the night to make sure his oxygen levels and breathing were in the normal range, his trach was getting the necessary humidity, and was clear of obstruction. They were also responsible for getting Walter up for the day, starting breathing treatments, and cleaning and sterilizing the equipment.

We had several different nurses in our home. The first day nurse ended up having to leave due to an emergency medical condition. We missed her. That was just the beginning of many more nurses that came and went for various reasons. Because of that, we had the opportunity to interview several nurses. We made nurse interviews a family affair. The entire family was impacted by the nurse's presence in our home; therefore, the family should be part of the interview process. We wanted Walter and Lydia to see the nurse candidate, interact, and give us their feedback. It was important because Walter would be with the nurse daily outside of our presence. If he didn't have good vibes, we listened. If we didn't feel the nurse was a good fit, we wouldn't hire her. The nursing agency would send a nurse to be interviewed by us to see if she would be a good fit. They knew we were particular, and at times they would do some pre-screening. Some of the questions we asked were:

- How far is your commute? Is your transportation reliable?
- How far away from home have you commuted for work?
- What nursing experience do you have?
- What trach experience do you have?
- Do you have children?
- How long have you worked for this agency or in-home care?
- Why did you choose home care nursing?
- Have you worked with an African American family before?

These questions allowed us to get a better understanding of the nurse's experience and nursing background. This also helped us understand somewhat their motivation for nursing and experience with children. We wanted to make sure the nurse was a good fit for Walter and the family.

We had the opportunity to set the boundaries for our home and how we wanted things to flow. There was constant dialogue and learning. We learned how to be employers and manage the nurses in our home. The main objective for the nurse was the care of our son. We kept it the number one priority

We definitely were not void of nursing stories, and we never had anything significant where Walter was in immediate danger. I remember coming home early from work one day, and the nurse was stretched out on my couch asleep. I had to release one nurse whom my son liked because she failed to remember her number one responsibility – my son's care. She put him in jeopardy, and I removed her to protect my son. Sometimes a nurse did not work out for our family. Sometimes our family or location did not work out for a nurse. We learned to be ok with it and how to adjust. I appreciated that I didn't have to explain why I would like to release a nurse to the nursing agency. This made it easier for me because I did not need a legitimate reason on a so-called list to remove a nurse nor remain in a negative situation. There were plenty of adventures, and we were fortunate to only release two nurses out of the many nurses we had.

Tips: Setting Boundaries in Your Home

Remember, your home is just that, your home. A nurse should not interrupt your home but complement it. The nurse should be trained; however, you can show her techniques for your child if necessary. You will have an opportunity to provide the nursing agency with the guidelines for your home. You will make the rules and are empowered to enforce them. Some guidelines should be gathered from you and shared with your nurse. A few are listed below:

- Parking
- Storage of nurse's items
- Nurse's location in your home (what space will they have in your home, facilities they use, etc.)
- Daily Activities/Family Schedule routine
- Expectations with school and teachers
- Use of Kitchen/appliances, etc.
- How to deal with siblings
- Disaster Planning (Fire, Tornado, etc.)

The Nursing Agency provided a form for us to complete that allowed us to detail instructions about Walter's care, which helped our home run smoothly because we had set boundaries. I have provided a list of questions that may be helpful as you establish boundaries in your home. There may also be other details to include for some of the things listed above, such as a disaster plan.

Setting Boundaries in the Home

(Example Questionnaire)

REGARDING THE CHILD:

Routines: What are your preferences regarding playtime, nap time, and bedtime? We realize such things impact the entire family. For example, if family members shower in the early morning, should the child be bathed at night? Does Mom like to bathe the child at times?

Meals/Snacks: Where will the child eat? Will the child eat with other family members while the nurse remains in another room, or should the nurse be present to feed the child?

Clothing: Who should choose the child's clothes for the day? If the nurse is to do so, please show them where the clothes are located. You may also want to tell them if you have a regular laundry day and advise when bed linens are to be changed.

Discipline: What is your philosophy of discipline concerning the child? Who administers it? What procedures should be followed in your absence?

REGARDING THE SIBLINGS:

Interactions: How and when will siblings interact with the child? What is the nurse's responsibility in supervising play?

Discipline: Do parents want nurses to intervene when siblings argue, or do they prefer the nurse to call them to address the problem?

Meals: Although nurses will provide their own meals, they need to know where perishables may be stored and where they may eat.

Television/Radio: Tell us whether nurses may use a TV or radio during the day and night hours. Consider that both are of help in remaining alert at night.

Telephone: Parents need to understand nurses may need to use the phone to make calls regarding the client. A nurse may make phone calls on behalf of the client.

Visitors: Who may enter the home to visit in the absence of parents? Is a list of names needed?

Participation In Care: How do family members want to participate in the child's care?

Communication: What information would you like to know right away? What can wait? For example, do you wish to be awakened if the child experiences a temperature elevation?

Privacy: Please tell us if there are particular times family members don't want to be disturbed?

REGARDING THE PARENTS:

Communication: What information should be reported to the parents immediately? What can wait? Do you want to set aside specific times to meet with each nurse?

Privacy: Please tell us if there are times when you don't want to be disturbed unless there is an extreme emergency. What else can the nursing staff do to preserve privacy in your family?

Chapter 8

Navigating School – 504/Individual Education (IEP) Plans

The school was another place to navigate. Walter was in first grade when he became critically ill, and his school year was interrupted. While he was hospitalized for nearly two months, I would bring worksheets from the school to keep him learning. We were very fortunate Walter had been in an advanced Kindergarten program where he had learned to read and do math which helped him not fall too far behind.

After coming home from the hospital, Walter was homeschooled by the school district. We chose to homeschool because he had stomach surgery scheduled for February. This allowed him and us to adjust at home and him to heal after surgery without another significant interruption in school. The homeschool teacher came to our house a few days during the week to work with him on his schoolwork. Walter wanted to return to school, so we allowed him to return after Spring Break, which was sufficient time after the stomach procedure. However, before he could safely return to school, we had to put a 504 Plan in place for him, which allowed accommodations due to illness and/or disability. Walter would always need to be accompanied by a nurse or trained caregiver at school. There were limitations for PE class and some school activities. Walter was always a very active child who played very hard. Slowing down wasn't the easiest thing for him; therefore, we trained him to listen to his body and stay hydrated. He successfully completed the school year physically, in-person April and May.

Before the beginning of each school year, I would contact the school office to request a 504 Plan meeting. In this meeting, the accommodations necessary for Walter's safety were discussed, agreed upon, and documented. In our experience, we've had the principal, school nurse, Walter's teachers, school social worker, guidance counselor, Walter's nurse, and our family in attendance. In one meeting early on, we even had a Bus Depot representative because he arranged for Walter's curb pick-up. Some of the accommodations we made were:

- A place for the nurse to be in continuous eyeshot of Walter.
- A safe and private place for Walter to have his trach suctioned and receive needed care.
- Allowing extra time for him to change classes. He could leave a couple of minutes earlier.

- Accommodate nurse on the school bus.
- Curbside pick-up and drop-off
- PE accommodations – participate as comfortable and avoid exercising outside in hot/cold weather.
- Asthma plan in place
- Ability to carry and drink bottled water during the day.
- No water play. No aerosol sprays/chalk powder.
- As Walter got into Junior/High School, we had a plan for any emergency care needs if an ambulance needed to be called to the school.

There were days when we accompanied Walter to school because there was a nursing conflict and no replacement. For us, school attendance was vital. If we did not have nursing coverage, Franklin or I went to school with Walter. At times, Franklin would come in from work in the morning, shower, and get dressed to accompany Walter to school. On other days, I would get dressed for school instead of work. At times, we would split the day. We did what was necessary to support his success in school. Those were some loooong days but so worth it. We got the opportunity to meet his teachers and see how he interacted with them and his peers. His teachers had the opportunity to provide feedback on Walter's behavior and schoolwork directly while we were there. Walter was almost always complimented on his polite and respectful behavior.

I made it a point to build a relationship with the school's nurse where Walter attended to ensure she knew who he was and what he needed. I wanted her to feel comfortable reaching out to me with any questions or concerns. I wanted her to know we were the parents and always had the final say concerning our child. I understood although a 504 Plan brought people together, it didn't build a relationship and rapport. The 504 Plan meetings would be a faint memory by the time of the first parent-teacher conference, and at times teachers changed during the school year. Therefore, it was necessary to build those relationships.

Tips: Partnering with schools for your child's education and safety

Although we only needed a 504 Plan in place for Walter's physical health needs, you may also need to put an Individual Education Plan (IEP) in place for your child if there are learning impairments. There are differences between the 504 Plan and the IEP. The 504 Plan shows how the school will support your child by removing or reducing barriers due to a disability. The 504 Plan will provide services to help students learn with their classmates. The IEP is a plan on how the school will meet any special educational needs. The IEP will create an individual learning plan to meet your child's unique needs. It will cover any of the disabilities listed in the Individuals with Disabilities Education Act (IDEA). I found a good source at www.understood.org explaining the difference between the 504 and IEP Plans.

Some of the tips I have about school are no different than any other child. But your child has some unique needs that require a little extra engagement.

- Be engaged. You are always the parent, even though they may see your child's nurse daily.
- Reach out to your child's teachers to let them know you are engaged and want to know how your child is doing.
- Get to know the school principal, your child's principal if separate, the school nurse, and the school secretary. Build a relationship, so they know you and your child.

- Make sure the teachers and school administrators understand that your child's nurse/caregiver is the first line of defense for your child's safety. If the nurse is not performing as expected (according to the 504 Plan), they should inform you, the parent. (I actually had to release a nurse my son liked because she sat in the building while my son was out for recess. When confronted by the school's nurse, she stated it was fine because she could see Walter on the field. The school nurse called me to inform me and said she was uncomfortable because there was no way to recognize if Walter was in distress or get to him quickly. That was not the first thing that I had to address with that nurse; however, it was the last.)
- Make it clear to your child's nurse what your expectation for school is. It is nice having an adult with your child daily, and it helps keep some of the distractions at bay. However, there needs to be a clear understanding and distinction between the nurse's job and yours as a parent. If the teacher has non-medical issues or questions about your child that need to be addressed, the teacher or the nurse should contact the parents.

Chapter 9

LIVE In Your New Normal

It takes time to build new routines and ways of doing things to make new grooves. It took us a few months to get into a new rhythm. ***Our entire life was impacted***. I remember, after Walter got his trach, we put family trips off that following year along with any thoughts of traveling any time in the near future. Franklin's mother and most of our families lived in the Southern United States, and we usually visited yearly. Walter was scheduled for reconstruction surgery in the summer of 2008, and all our hopes were on it as our ticket back to 'normal.' We were hoping the surgery would fix his airway, and he wouldn't need the trach tube anymore. But, we didn't know how long he would need the trach. I was in a 'wait until after' mindset. One day, during my quiet time, these questions hit me: *What are you waiting for? Why are you putting your life on hold? What if Walter is never able to breathe without the trach? Are you going to just wait?*

I had to make a choice – continue to wait, for however long, or find a way to LIVE in the 'New Normal' we were thrust into. *I decided to LIVE now!* I am glad I made that decision because Walter was trach-dependent for 8 years, 2 months, and 14 days.

Tips: My final tips will help you *LIVE* in your New Normal.

Give yourself and your family time to adjust to the new normal. It is a new world. You are not only a parent but a caregiver, advocate, and employer. You have nurses in your home and plenty of doctor's appointments to color your calendar. ***But, LIVE in your new normal!*** **LIVE** within your boundaries; don't allow your boundaries to be your life. Don't wait until _____ happens. You fill in the blank. It may never happen. Don't let precious time pass you by. **LIVE!**.

Take Care of You: Being a parent is hard work. Adding the role of caregiver brings another level of duty to that, so taking care of you in the midst of it is crucial. In our situation, Walter was required to always be with a trained caregiver. If he was not with a nurse, he was with at least one of us. So, it was necessary to find ways to get a breather. If you've ever flown on an airplane, one of the first things that happen at the start of the flight is the flight attendant shares the seatbelt and safety protocol. She says, "If the plane loses oxygen in the cabin, an oxygen mask will drop. If you are with children, please put it on yourself <u>before</u> you put it on your child." **IT IS IMPERATIVE FOR YOU, THE PARENT and CAREGIVER**, to get the necessary oxygen to be well enough to take care of your child. If ***<u>YOU</u>*** are not ok, your child or children will not be ok. A few things I suggest are:

- *Train someone else you trust to care for your child.* Walter's godmother trained with us, which enabled us to have someone in place in case of emergency or just when we needed a break.
- *Maintain a personal quiet time/meditate.* Having quiet time to spend alone with the Word of God and in prayer helped to keep me centered and focused. It gave me strength when I felt like I was overwhelmed.
- *Spend time with your friends and family.* We are people of faith. I spent time in my women's group activities, and my husband had times of fellowship with his men's group. We also invited others over to fill our home with love and laughter. It not only helped us, but the children also enjoyed it too. Believe me; you both will need a break from the normal routine.
- *Take a specific time, each quarter if possible, of the year to focus on you.* Just having those times to look forward to will tremendously help you mentally and physically. It could be a night in a hotel or a day away to do something you enjoy. It could be alone, with friends, or your spouse. Make your time a priority.
- *Join a support group.* Although I didn't know of any support groups when we started our journey, there are many Tracheostomy support groups on Facebook now.

Take Care of Your Marriage: One of the tougher things to do when you begin to have children is to keep your marriage relationship growing. Well, when you have a child with critical health concerns, another level of intentionality is needed. You have to find time for you and your spouse to connect – talk, touch, and be intimate. Bringing Walter home this time was like bringing a new baby home – adjusting to caring for him on our own, recognizing what he needs, and responding confidently. *It is imperative you and your spouse remain connected on this journey because you need each other. You are a team.*

Honestly…. we struggled. It was only the grace of God and our commitment to Him that helped us remain attached. Please take these simple suggestions to help you stay connected, as you will be tested. Each of you will process your journey differently, and you must be committed to staying connected.

It will be more challenging to physically get away; so, take advantage of the time you do have instead of focusing on what you no longer can do without extensive coordination. Keep it simple and manage what you can control.

- *Movie Night*: Rent or stream a movie to watch with your spouse for a date night. Use your creativity to make it fun.
- *Candlelight dinner*: Create your own special time of intimacy.
- *Dance*: Put on some music and dance together.
- *Coffee/Tea time:* Create and keep an opportunity to talk with each other about everything household-related. Make sure it's a time that works for both of you.
- *Talk time*: Set aside a specific time, whenever it works for you, to focus on and talk about your relationship.
- *Plan for the more significant celebrations*: For birthdays, wedding anniversaries, marriage weekend retreats, or special occasions, get additional care scheduled ahead of time. Make reservations early. We would alternate with Walter's godparents to attend our Marriage Retreats.

They would stay and keep our children for the weekend while we participated in the retreat, and then the following year, they would go. This helped to give us <u>all</u> the needed time. The kids got a break from us and us from them. On top of that, the godparents got precious time to spend with the kids.

Take Care of Your Family: It was important for Walter to attend school regularly, my husband and I to work, and to have time alone as a family. Therefore, we used the skilled nursing hours we were awarded to support those priorities.

Find ways to do some of the things you enjoy as a family - family vacations, road trips, or what you prefer. We didn't allow Walter to stay focused on what he could no longer do but to focus on what he **COULD** do.

Coming into his first summer with the trach, he said to me, *"Mom, I won't be able to swim anymore.*

I said, "Well, could you swim before the trach?"

He said, "No."

Then I followed up with, "Well, you won't miss it then. You can still play in the water, but you just can't go under the water nor put yourself in a situation where water can get into your trach. You can drown if you do."

That was the last "I can't" conversation we had. Walter played on the rec basketball team, won trophies in his bowling league, went to summer day camp, and even played the clarinet with a trach. So, there is life with a trach. LIVE within the limitations! **Don't let the limitations be your life.**

After deciding to LIVE now, I found out how to continue to go on family trips and vacations. I booked a spring break trip to Branson, Missouri. It was about 7 hours from our home, and it was a great test before traveling 12-14 hours to visit family. We had Walter's oxygen delivered to the hotel where we would stay. The medical supply company we had at that time was nationwide. They could deliver equipment to locations across the country if it was within a certain distance within that state. When we got to the hotel, the equipment was there waiting on us. The vacation was a little different, but we thoroughly enjoyed it! We continued to travel and visit family as we had previously done, happily within our New Normal boundaries.

Siblings & friends: One thing to be cautious of is allowing your energy and focus to always be on the special-needs child or the well-child. **All your children need your attention. You must celebrate each child's accomplishments.** Their individual abilities are different; therefore, they require different rewards and expressions of appreciation. Teach them how to celebrate each other by attending events for them and bringing the other children along. Celebrate their successes. This will help them learn how to celebrate each other's successes.

One of the things I've always done is make birthdays a big deal. When the children wake up, there are balloons, a happy birthday banner, and decorations. The day includes their favorite meal, dessert, and gifts. The birthday celebrations almost always had birthday parties, especially at 1, 5, 10, 13, and 16, with smaller playdates or hangouts with a friend or two for the other ages. This is a simple way to make each child feel special.

Because Walter could not have sleepovers at his friends' houses, we would allow sleepovers and playdates at our home. Some Saturdays, I would pick up some of their friends, go to McDonald's or the park, and just let them play for hours and then grab lunch. We would do movie playdates while I struggled to keep from dozing off in the middle of it. We knew how vital bonding with friends and having time with their age group was for their social development. So, we wanted them to have that opportunity to experience being a kid and enjoying childhood.

Capture the memories: Sometimes, as parents, we can be so in the thick of being a caregiver that we forget the children are growing up. **Take pictures all along the way. Take pictures of the good, the bad, and the ugly.** The photos are the testimony of your experience and life. They help you remember what life causes you to forget. I took pictures of my son in the hospital, at home, and everywhere else. We captured birthday celebrations, playdates, riding in the car, and just sitting. Make the memories and capture the moments. You will be able to look back at how blessed you are and be grateful for making it through the various challenges of life.

LIVE in the moment, don't worry: This may be easier said than done, but enjoy the journey along the way. Each day will bring its answers and troubles, but you will only be able to live each moment as it comes. Plan ahead, but LIVE in each moment. All my worries and questions eventually were answered. We financially managed Walter's care through insurance from our employers, supplemented by a state-sponsored program for critically ill children, which paid for nursing hours. We eventually sold our other house and got back to one mortgage. We were able to care for Walter at home successfully and did a great job. Walter did well in school and did not get behind. I heard Walter's laughs again with the help of the Passy Muir Speaking Valve, which forced air over the vocal cords and through the mouth for a stronger, less breathy voice. **By the grace of God, I learned that we were stronger than we had believed and had become more resilient through this experience.**

Develop Your Plan

I know your story most likely is different from ours, but I'm sure there are some things you can do to create a New Normal for you and your family. Here are some questions and thoughts that may help you determine how you want to live. Use the blank note pages as your scratch paper to develop your plan of approach.

1. What do I enjoy doing that helps me relax?
2. Am I taking care of myself? What is my body trying to tell me?
3. What are the things my family value? What are the most important things to us as a family?
4. What does my family enjoy doing together? Do we need to do it differently now? How can we continue to do it?
5. What do my spouse/partner and I enjoy doing together? Are there any changes we need to consider?
6. Who are others I trust and think would be responsible enough to train and care for my special child/children?
7. What sibling rivalry am I noticing due to the additional care needed for my child? What honest crucial and critical conversations will I have to ensure all are getting what they need?
8. What other questions do I have? Are there any other specific items I need to address?

Determine How You Will LIVE In Your New Normal

What new things will you do?

_____
_____
_____
_____

What will you do differently?

_____
_____
_____
_____

Notes

Notes

Notes

References:

1. "How does a Tracheostomy Tube Work" Image, 2004-2020 www.AboutKidsHealth.ca
2. "Signs of Respiratory Distress," https://www.hopkinsmedicine.org/health/conditions-and-diseases/signs-of-respiratory-distress
3. "The Difference Between IEPs and 504 Plans", The Understood Team, Andrew M.I. Lee, JD - Reviewer, https://www.understood.org/en/school-learning/special-services/504-plan/the-difference-between-ieps-and-504-plans (The Understood Team, Andrew M.I. Lee, JD –Reviewer)

Leave A Review

Were you encouraged by this book?

Don't forget to leave a review!

Every review matters, and it matters a *lot!*

Head on over and leave a review on Amazon.com.

Send any specific inquiries about the book to

info.melbashareshope@gmail.com

I thank you endlessly.

Read More!

If you would like to read more from this author, go to **www.melbashareshope.com** and download:

While You Wait

If you would like to dive a little deeper into Melba's story, keep your eyes open for her next book:

The Miracle of the Meantime

About the Author

Melba K. Haggins is a calming force in the middle of a storm. Her words quiet the storm and provide others with hope in an ever-changing world. Although she has had her share of hardships and life challenges, they have strengthened her relationship and faith in God, which has enabled her and her family to be overcomers. Her confidence in God gives her the grace to walk in love, wisdom, faith, and courage in the face of chaos to produce change.

Mrs. Haggins is a servant-leader and gifted teacher. Her teaching gift is undeniable. She can ignite one's passion to pursue their God-given purpose and understand their true identity. She has served in the local church for over 40 years in various capacities and currently as a licensed minister. She is also a highly trained Information Technology Professional and has served nearly 20 years as a skilled team leader. To serve and give back to the community, in 2008, she and her family started an initiative called "Spread the Hope." This effort supports families whose children are hospitalized, something the Haggins family knew all too well.

She earned a bachelor's degree in Computer Science from Grambling State University, a Master's in Business Administration (MBA) from the University of Louisiana at

Monroe (formerly, Northeast Louisiana University), and a bachelor's degree in Theology from Life Christian University, along with several other professional certifications and designations.

Born and raised in Louisiana and currently residing in Central Illinois, Melba is a devoted wife and mother. She takes extreme pleasure in seeing her children and others grow, learn and pursue their God-given passions and dreams. Mrs. Haggins enjoys learning, traveling, cooking, performing arts, and spending quality time with family and friends. She often shares her story of faith to give hope to those who feel overwhelmed by life and its challenges. Melba K. Haggins has stood the test of time and is known to be unshakeable in the face of adversity. One of her favorite scriptures states, "Faithful is He who calleth you, who also will do it" (*I Thessalonians 5:24 KJV*). This woman is proof to the world that God will do exactly what He said.

Melba is available for:

Professional and Ministry Workshops & Conferences, Leadership Training & Development, Team-Building, Facilitation, and Interviews

Contact Information:

Email – info.melbashareshope@gmail.com

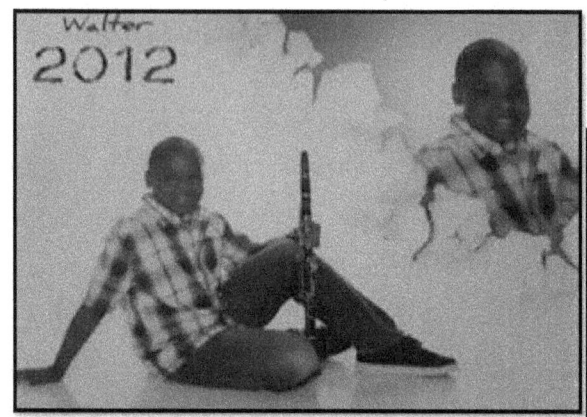
← Walter plays clarinet

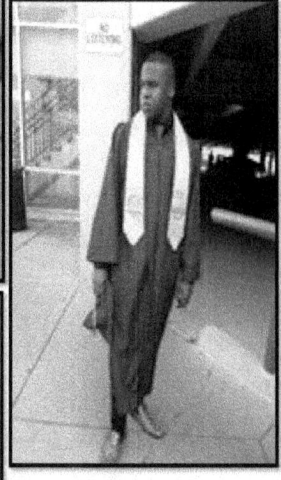

High School Graduation

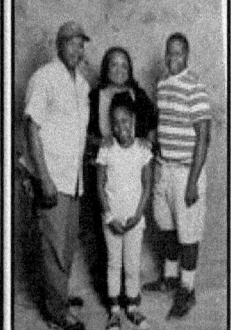
← Family Snapshots

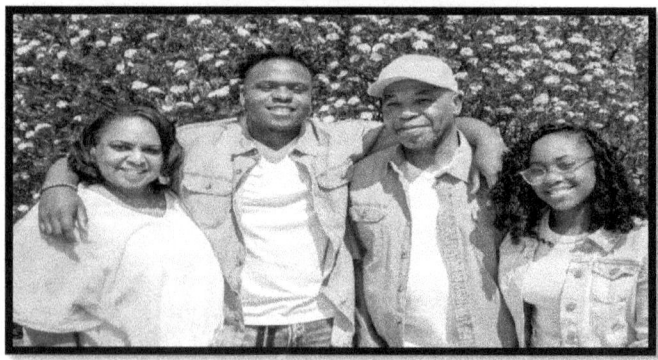

www.ingramcontent.com/pod-product-compliance
Lightning Source LLC
Chambersburg PA
CBHW070326100426
42743CB00011B/2578